59 CASTOR OIL RECIPES FOR HEALTHY LIVING

The Ultimate Secret Remedies for Unleashing and Harnessing Nature's Elixirs for Hair Growth, Eyelashes and Smooth Skin

Marie A. Heavener

TABLE OF CONTENT

INTRODUCTION

Tamika lives in a vibrant city. Tamika appeared to have everything, from an infectious grin to a heart full of hope. Despite her pleasant demeanor, she fought silently with her anxieties.

The mirror did not reflect the lively, confident woman she intended to be, but rather one afflicted by the constant troubles of hair loss, poor skin tone, and sparse lashes.

These hardships have shaped Tamika's life. Each day brought a new wave of despair as she saw her once-luscious hair fade and her complexion lose its natural radiance.

The reflection looking back at her seemed like a harsh mocking of the vibrant soul she had within.

Tamika found herself crawling into the shadows during public occasions, afflicted by acute shyness caused by her lack of confidence in her physical appearance. The fear of criticism hung over her like a black cloud, suffocating her capacity to express herself freely and live life to the utmost.

Despite the despair, a ray of hope appeared in the form of a book, a treasure trove of information and sustenance that would become her beacon of light in the darkest of times. Within its pages is a compilation of recipes thoughtfully prepared to nourish both the body and the soul.

With resolve in her heart, Tamika set out on a voyage of self-discovery, equipped with the transformational power of these recipes. Each recipe became a monument to her unrelenting will to restore her health and vigor.

Tamika saw a stunning shift within herself as the weeks evolved into months. Her previously drab strands of hair began to regain their former power and luster, and her complexion flowered with a renewed brilliance that appeared to defy age and adversity.

Even her lashes, which were previously thin and uninteresting, now surrounded her eyes with a compelling charm that said volumes about her inner beauty.

Perhaps the most significant shift was Tamika's newfound confidence, which emanated from her very essence. She no longer avoided the spotlight but welcomed it with wide arms, relishing the opportunity to express herself openly and unapologetically.

Tamika is now living her best life, free of her prior anxieties. Thanks to the insight taught by this book, her fears and anxiety about frequent hair loss and a mediocre look are distant memories, eclipsed by the bright glow of her regained vigor and self-confidence.

HOW TO USE THIS BOOK

Castor Oil Recipes for Healthy Living" is a thorough manual that digs into the many advantages of castor oil for beauty and overall well-being.

From nourishing beautiful locks to creating bright skin and enticing eyelashes, this book is an excellent resource for anybody looking for natural and efficient beauty remedies.

The book begins by explaining the extraordinary qualities of castor oil, emphasizing its high concentration of fatty acids, vitamins, and minerals that nourish and revitalize the hair, skin, and lashes.

You will be presented with the science underlying castor oil's usefulness, allowing you to make more educated decisions regarding your beauty regimen.

With a user-friendly approach, this book covers a varied range of recipes and procedures adapted to individual beauty needs.

For hair development, you will learn about rejuvenating scalp treatments, hair masks, and massage methods that stimulate circulation, strengthen follicles, and promote healthy growth. Also you will understand the use of castor oil as a natural treatment for common scalp disorders such as dandruff and itching.

In terms of skincare, you will be treated to exquisite face cleansers, moisturizers, and serums enriched with castor oil to encourage smooth, supple skin and reduce the appearance of fine lines and wrinkles.

This book delves into the therapeutic benefits of castor oil for treating acne, scars, and other dermatological concerns, providing mild yet effective solutions for reaching a beautiful complexion.

One of this book's notable aspects is in the recipes on how to improve eyelash health and attractiveness. You will discover new ways to apply castor oil to your lashes, boosting growth, thickness, and length for fluttery, appealing eyes.

Each recipe in the book is accompanied by practical step-by-step directions, and enlightening benefits , ensuring that read
you can easily and confidently include castor oil into your daily beauty regimen.

Whether you want to renew dull hair, rejuvenate weary skin, or increase the attractiveness of eyelashes,the Castor Oil Recipes in this book covers problems affecting Hair Growth, Smooth Skin, and Eyelashes there by providing a wealth of information and inspiration for maximizing the benefits of castor oil in beauty care.

CASTOR OIL RECIPES FOR UNLEASHING YOUR BEAUTY AND CHARMING LOOKS

1. Castor Oil Hair Growth Mask

Ingredients:

2 tablespoons of castor oil.

1 tablespoon of coconut oil.

1 tablespoon honey.

Preparation:

In a mixing dish, combine all of the ingredients thoroughly.

into your scalp and hair,the mixture should be gently massaged

Leave it on for 30-60 minutes.

Rinse well with shampoo and warm water.

Benefits:

It promotes thick hair development by feeding the scalp and hair follicles.

Conditions the hair, making it smoother and easier to maintain.

Reduces hair breakage and split ends, resulting in healthier hair overall.

2. *Castor Oil and Aloe Vera Skin Moisturizer*

Ingredients:

2 tablespoons of castor oil.

2 teaspoons of aloe vera gel.

1 tablespoon Shea butter

Preparation:

Combine all of the ingredients in a mixing bowl.

Until you achieve a smooth creamy consistency, don't stop Mixing thoroughly.

Apply the moisturizer to your skin, concentrating on the dry areas.

Massage gently until completely absorbed.

Benefits:

By making the Skin supple and smooth,it nourishes and hydrates the skin

Relieves inflammation and soothes inflamed skin.

Improves skin elasticity and gives a more youthful look.

3. Castor Oil Eyelash Serum

Ingredients:

1 teaspoon of castor oil.

1 teaspoon of sweet almond oil.

1 teaspoon of vitamin E oil.

Preparation:

Combine all of the oils in a clean container.

Before going to bed, apply the serum to your lashes with a clean mascara wand or cotton swab.

Leave it on overnight.

Rinse gently with lukewarm water in the morning.

Benefits:

Encourages eyelash development, making them longer and thicker.

Conditions and strengthens eyelashes, preventing breakage.

Moisturizes the eyelashes and keeps them from getting brittle.

4. Castor Oil and Brown Sugar Body Scrub

Ingredients:

2 tablespoons of castor oil.

1/4 cup brown sugar.

1 tablespoon honey.

Preparation:

In a mixing basin, combine the castor oil, brown sugar, and honey until thoroughly blended.

Apply the mixture to moist skin in the shower, working in circular movements.

for a few minutes,gently exfoliate your skin

Rinse well with warm water.

Benefits:

Exfoliation removes dead skin cells, exposing smoother, healthier skin.

Moisturizes the skin, making it smooth and supple.

Improves blood circulation, resulting in a bright complexion.

5. Castor Oil Hair Serum

Ingredients:

2 tablespoons of castor oil.

1 tablespoon of argan oil.

5 drops of lavender essential oil.

Preparation:

Combine all of the oils in a tiny glass container.

Shake well to combine the ingredients.

Apply a few drops of the serum to the ends of your hair, not the scalp.

Allow it to sit overnight or for at least a few hours before washing.

Benefits:

Nourishes and strengthens the hair, minimizing breakage and split ends.

Adds sheen and sparkle to the hair, making it seem healthier.

By resulting in a more manageable and smoother hair,it helps to reduce frizz and flyaways,

6. Castor Oil and Turmeric Face Mask

Ingredients:

1 tablespoon of castor oil.

1/2 teaspoon of turmeric powder.

One spoonful of yogurt

Preparation:

In a small bowl, combine the castor oil, turmeric powder, and yogurt until smooth.

Use the mixture on clean, dry skin, avoiding the eyes.

Leave it on for around 15-20 minutes.

Rinse with lukewarm water, then pat dry.

Benefits:

Turmeric contains anti-inflammatory qualities that can help treat acne and soothe inflamed skin.

Castor oil intensely hydrates the skin, making it smooth and supple.

Yogurt contains lactic acid, which gently exfoliates the skin, revealing a more vibrant complexion.

7. Castor Oil Hair Growth Serum

Ingredients:

2 tablespoons of castor oil.

1 tablespoon of jojoba oil.

5 drops of rosemary essential oil.

Preparation:

Combine all of the oils in a tiny glass dropper container.

Shake vigorously to combine the ingredients well.

Apply a few drops of serum to your scalp and gently massage it.

Leave it on overnight and wash it off in the morning with a gentle shampoo.

Benefits:

Stimulates hair follicles, promoting thicker and healthier hair growth.

Jojoba oil hydrates the scalp and helps to control sebum production.

Rosemary essential oil stimulates blood circulation to the scalp, which promotes hair growth.

8. Castor Oil Lip Balm

Ingredients:

1 tablespoon of castor oil.

1 tablespoon of beeswax pellets.

1 teaspoon honey.

3-4 drops of peppermint essential oil (optional for taste).

Preparation:

In a double boiler, combine the castor oil and beeswax pellets at low heat.

When melted, remove from heat and whisk in honey and peppermint oil (if desired).

Pour the liquid into tiny lip balm containers and allow to cool and set.

Benefits:

Castor oil hydrates and nourishes the lips, leaving them smooth and moisturized.

Beeswax creates a protective layer around the lips, limiting moisture loss.

Honey contains antibacterial qualities that cure and prevent damaged lips.

9. Castor Oil and Green Tea Facial Toner

Ingredients:

1/2 cup brewed green tea, chilled.

1 tablespoon of witch hazel.

1 tablespoon of castor oil.

Preparation:

In a clean container, mix cooled green tea, witch hazel, and castor oil.

Shake well to completely combine all of the ingredients.

After cleaning your skin, use the toner with a cotton pad, concentrating on oily areas.

Let it air dry before adding moisturizer.

Benefits:

Green tea is high in antioxidants, which fight free radicals and decrease inflammation.

Witch hazel is an astringent, which tightens pores and reduces excess oil production.

Castor oil hydrates without blocking pores, leaving the skin feeling balanced and revitalized.

10. Castor oil and oatmeal bath soak

Ingredients:

1/2 cup colloidal oatmeal.

2 tablespoons castor oil

5 drops of lavender essential oil.

Preparation:

In a mixing dish, blend the colloidal oatmeal, castor oil, and lavender essential oil until thoroughly incorporated.

Fill your bathtub with warm water and add the oatmeal mixture while it is running.

Stir the water to properly distribute the ingredients.

Soak in the bath for 15-20 minutes, then rinse with fresh water.

Benefits:

Colloidal oatmeal relieves dry, itchy skin while also reducing minor irritations and inflammation.

Castor oil significantly hydrates the skin, making it smooth and moisturized.

Lavender essential oil has a relaxing impact on both the mind and body, encouraging relaxation and stress alleviation.

11. Castor Oil Hair Growth Scalp Massage Oil.

Ingredients:

2 tablespoons of castor oil.

1 tablespoon of olive oil.

5 drops of peppermint essential oil.

Preparation:

Combine the castor oil, olive oil, and peppermint essential oil in a small mixing basin.

To improve oil absorption, gently heat the mixture for a few seconds.

Apply heated oil to your scalp and gently massage for 5-10 minutes.

Before shampooing your hair,Leave it on for at least 30 minutes

Benefits:

Castor oil nourishes the scalp and strengthens hair follicles, hence stimulating hair growth.

Olive oil moisturizes the scalp and helps prevent dandruff.

Peppermint essential oil improves blood circulation in the scalp, which promotes hair growth.

12. Castor Oil and Shea Butter Hand Cream.

Ingredients:

2 tablespoons of castor oil

2 tablespoons of shea butter

1 tablespoon of coconut oil.

5 drops of your preferred essential oil (optional).

Preparation:

In a double boiler, combine the castor oil, shea butter, and coconut oil over low heat.

Allow it to cool slightly after removing it from the the heat source once it has melted

Stir in your preferred essential oil for aroma (if using).

Transfer the mixture to a clean container and let it harden.

Benefits:

Castor oil gives great hydration and heals dry and broken skin on the hands.

Shea butter is high in vitamins and fatty acids, which nourish and soften the skin.

Coconut oil retains moisture and creates a protective barrier, reducing moisture loss.

13. Castor Oil and Lemon Lip Scrub.

Ingredients:

1 tablespoon of castor oil.

1 tablespoon of granulated sugar.

1 teaspoon of lemon juice.

Preparation:

In a small bowl, blend the castor oil, granulated sugar, and lemon juice until thoroughly incorporated.

Massage the mixture onto your lips in circular movements for around 1-2 minutes.

Rinse with lukewarm water, then pat dry.

Apply a hydrating lip balm next.

Benefits:

Castor oil thoroughly hydrates the lips, keeping them from becoming dry and chapped.

Sugar exfoliates dead skin cells, resulting in smoother, softer lips.

Lemon juice brightens the lips and helps to reduce dark patches or discoloration.

14. Castor Oil and Avocado Hair Mask.

Ingredients:

1 ripe avocado.

2 tablespoons of castor oil.

1 tablespoon honey.

Preparation:

In a mixing basin, mash the ripe avocado until completely smooth.

Combine the castor oil and honey with the mashed avocado and stir thoroughly.

Apply the mixture to moist hair, concentrating on the roots and tips.

Leave it on for 30 to 60 minutes, then rinse with shampoo and water.

Benefits:

Avocado nourishes and strengthens the hair, boosting growth and avoiding damage.

Castor oil improves blood circulation in the scalp, which promotes healthy hair growth.

Honey is a humectant, which attracts and seals in moisture, leaving the hair smooth and nourished.

15 Castor Oil and Tea Tree Oil Acne Spot Treatment.

Ingredients:

1 tablespoon of castor oil.

3-4 drops of tea tree essential oil

Preparation:

Combine castor oil and tea tree essential oil in a small, clean container.

Use a cotton swab to apply the mixture directly to acne areas.

Leave it on overnight.

Rinse with lukewarm water in the morning.

Benefits:

Castor oil can help to lessen the irritation and redness associated with acne.

Tea tree oil contains antibacterial qualities that assist to fight acne-causing germs.

Together, these oils help hasten the healing process of acne patches, resulting in cleaner skin.

16. Castor Oil and Rosehip Seed Oil Facial Serum.

Ingredients:

1 tablespoon of castor oil.

1 tablespoon of rosehip seed oil.

3 drops of lavender essential oil (optional).

Preparation:

Combine the castor oil and rosehip seed oil in a small glass container.

If you want to add more aroma and tranquility, use lavender essential oil.

Shake thoroughly to mix all of the ingredients.

Apply a few drops of the serum to your clean, wet skin and gently massage in circular movements.

Benefits:

Castor oil thoroughly hydrates and nourishes the skin, minimizing dryness and flakiness.

Rosehip seed oil is high in vitamins A and C, which stimulate collagen formation and enhance skin suppleness.

The lavender essential oil contains relaxing effects that can help to relieve tension and soothe irritable skin.

17. Castor Oil and Cocoa Butter Body Lotion.

Ingredients:

2 tablespoons of castor oil.

2 tablespoons cocoa butter.

1 tablespoon of coconut oil.

5 drops of vanilla essential oil (optional).

Preparation:

In a double boiler, combine the castor oil, cocoa butter, and coconut oil over low heat.

Allow it to cool slightly after removing it from the heat source once it has melted

If desired, add vanilla essential oil for scent and thoroughly whisk.

Transfer the mixture to a clean container and let it harden.

Benefits:

Castor oil intensely hydrates the skin, making it smooth and supple.

Cocoa butter is high in antioxidants and fatty acids, which assist in enhancing skin suppleness and minimize the appearance of scars and stretch marks.

Coconut oil moisturizes and nourishes the skin, offering long-term hydration and protection.

18. Castor Oil and Cucumber Eye Gel

Ingredients:

1 tablespoon of castor oil.

1/4 cup cucumber juice (made from freshly shredded cucumber).

1 tablespoon of aloe vera gel.

Preparation:

In a blender, puree the shredded cucumber until smooth.

Strain the cucumber juice through a fine mesh screen to remove any pulp.

In a small dish, blend the castor oil, cucumber juice, and aloe vera gel until well-mixed.

Transfer the mixture to a clean container and chill for 30 minutes before using.

Benefits:

Castor oil nourishes and hydrates the sensitive skin around the eyes, minimizing the appearance of fine lines and wrinkles.

Cucumber juice contains cooling and relaxing characteristics, which can help decrease puffiness and dark circles under the eyes.

Aloe vera gel moisturizes and soothes the skin, offering relief from irritation and inflammation.

19. Castor Oil and Chamomile Facial Steam.

Ingredients:

1 tablespoon of castor oil.

2 cups of hot water.

1/4 cup dried chamomile flowers.

Preparation:

Put the dried chamomile flowers in a big basin.

Pour the boiling water over the chamomile flowers and wrap the basin with a cloth.

Allow the mixture to steep for 5-10 minutes to extract the chamomile's benefits.

Add the castor oil to the basin and mix thoroughly.

Lean over the bowl and place a cloth over your head to capture the steam.

Close your eyes and take deep breaths for 5-10 minutes.

Benefits:

Castor oil hydrates and nourishes the skin, making it smooth and moisturized.

Chamomile contains anti-inflammatory and calming qualities that assist in relieving inflamed skin and minimizing redness.

Facial steaming opens pores, allowing castor oil and chamomile to go deeper into the skin and provide optimum benefits.

20. *Castor Oil and Eucalyptus Hair Growth Treatment*

Ingredients:

2 tablespoons of castor oil.

1 tablespoon of eucalyptus essential oil.

1 tablespoon of olive oil.

Preparation:

In a small bowl, whisk together all of the oils until thoroughly blended.

For a few seconds and in a microwave Heat the mixture

Apply heated oil to your scalp and gently massage for 5-10 minutes.

before washing as usual,Let it sit for at least 30 minutes

Benefits:

Castor oil stimulates hair growth by feeding the scalp and strengthening the follicles.

Eucalyptus essential oil improves blood circulation in the scalp, which promotes hair growth.

Olive oil hydrates and nourishes hair, making it smooth and manageable while avoiding dryness and breakage.

21. Castor Oil and Almond Milk Bath Soak

Ingredients:

1/2 cup almond milk.

2 tablespoons of castor oil.

Add 1/4 cup of Epsom salt and 5 drops of lavender essential oil (optional).

Preparation:

Fill a bathtub with warm water and add almond milk, castor oil, and Epsom salt.

Add a few drops of lavender essential oil for a relaxing scent.

Stir the mixture thoroughly to achieve equitable distribution.

Soak in the bath for 20-30 minutes, then rinse with fresh water.

Benefits:

Almond milk provides vitamins and minerals that nourish and moisturize the skin.

Castor oil deeply hydrates the skin, leaving it hydrated and supple.

Epsom salt relaxes muscles, relieves pains, and detoxifies the skin, improving general well-being.

22. *Castor Oil and Grapefruit Lip Balm*

Ingredients:

1 tablespoon of castor oil.

1 tablespoon of beeswax pellets.

1 teaspoon of grapefruit zest.

3-4 drops of grapefruit essential oil.

Preparation:

In a double boiler, combine the castor oil and beeswax pellets at low heat.

Mix in the grapefruit zest and essential oil.

Pour the liquid into lip balm containers and allow it to cool and harden.

Benefits:

Castor oil gently hydrates and nourishes the lips, leaving them smooth and moisturized.

Beeswax creates a protective layer around the lips, limiting moisture loss.

Grapefruit essential oil has a pleasant smell and includes antioxidants, which encourage healthy-looking lips.

23. Castor Oil and Honey Face Mask

Ingredients:

1 tablespoon of castor oil.

1 tablespoon of raw honey.

1 teaspoon of lemon juice.

Preparation:

In a small bowl, whisk together the castor oil, honey, and lemon juice until thoroughly blended.

Use the mixture on clean, dry skin, avoiding the eyes.

For the next 15 to 20 minutes,Leave the mask on

Rinse with lukewarm water, then pat dry.

Benefits:

Castor oil intensely hydrates and nourishes the skin, making it smooth and supple.

Honey contains antimicrobial characteristics that can help treat acne and prevent outbreaks.

Lemon juice contains citric acid, which gently exfoliates and brightens the face.

24. *Castor Oil and Peppermint Foot Scrub*

Ingredients:

2 tablespoons of castor oil.

1/4 cup granulated sugar.

1 tablespoon of coconut oil.

5 drops of peppermint essential oil.

Preparation:

In a dish, blend the castor oil, granulated sugar, coconut oil, and peppermint essential oil until thoroughly mixed.

Wet your feet and apply the scrub, concentrating on tough regions such as heels and soles.

For a few minutes,and in circular strokes Massage gentle

Rinse with warm water, then pat dry.

Benefits:

Castor oil hydrates and nourishes dry, cracked heels, resulting in soft, smooth feet.

Sugar exfoliates dead skin cells, resulting in softer, healthier-looking feet.

Peppermint essential oil cools and soothes sore feet while also giving a pleasant scent.

25. *Castor Oil and Avocado Hair Conditioner*

Ingredients:

1 ripe avocado.

2 tablespoons of castor oil.

1 tablespoon honey.

Preparation:

In a mixing basin, mash the ripe avocado until completely smooth.

Combine the castor oil and honey with the mashed avocado and stir thoroughly.

Apply the mixture to moist hair, concentrating on the ends.

After 20-30 minutes, rinse completely with water.

Benefits:

Avocado thoroughly hydrates and nourishes hair, eliminating dryness and frizz.

Castor oil strengthens the hair shaft, promoting healthy hair growth.

Honey provides gloss and sparkle to your hair while also giving hydration.

26. Castor oil and lavender bath salts

Ingredients:

1 cup of Epsom salt.

2 tablespoons of castor oil.

Ten drops of lavender essential oil.

Preparation:

In a dish, mix the Epsom salt, castor oil, and lavender essential oil.

Mix well until the oils are uniformly dispersed.

Keep the bath salts in an airtight container until ready to use.

Benefits:

Epsom salt helps to relax muscles and relieve tension in the body.

Castor oil hydrates and softens the skin, making it smooth and moisturized.

Lavender essential oil promotes relaxation and reduces tension, resulting in a soothing bath experience.

27. Castor Oil and Coconut Milk Hair Mask

Ingredients:

2 tablespoons of castor oil.

1/4 cup coconut milk.

1 tablespoon honey.

Preparation:

In a dish, combine the castor oil, coconut milk, and honey.

Apply the mixture to damp hair, beginning at the roots and progressing to the ends.

For the next 30-60 minutes, let the mask sit, and also Cover your hair with a shower cap

Rinse well with warm water and apply shampoo as normal.

Benefits:

Castor oil benefits the scalp and encourages healthy hair development.

Coconut milk contains vitamins and minerals that strengthen hair and prevent damage.

Honey gives moisture to hair, making it silky, smooth, and manageable.

28. Castor Oil and Green Clay Face Mask

Ingredients:

1 tablespoon of castor oil.

1 spoonful of green clay.

1 tablespoon of apple cider vinegar.

1 teaspoon water (optional for consistency).

Preparation:

In a dish, combine the castor oil, green clay, and apple cider vinegar until a homogeneous paste develops.

If the mixture is too thick, gradually add water until the appropriate consistency is achieved.

Use the mask on clean, dry skin, avoiding the eye region.

Rinse with warm water after leaving it on for about 10-15 minutes

Benefits:

Castor oil moisturizes and nourishes the skin, making it smooth and supple.

Green clay removes excess oil and pollutants from the skin, detoxifying and clarifying pores.

Apple cider vinegar regulates the skin's pH and reduces irritation and redness.

29. *Castor Oil and Banana Hair Mask*

Ingredients:

1 ripe banana.

2 tablespoons of castor oil.

1 spoonful of yogurt

Preparation:

In a mixing bowl, mash the ripe banana until it is smooth.

Combine the castor oil and yogurt with the mashed banana and stir thoroughly.

Apply the mixture to moist hair, concentrating on the roots and tips.

For the next 30-60 minutes, let the mask sit, and also Cover your hair with a shower cap

Rinse well with warm water and apply shampoo as normal.

Benefits:

Castor oil benefits the scalp and encourages healthy hair development.

Bananas are high in vitamins and minerals, which help to strengthen and elasticity your hair.
Yogurt contains lactic acid, which cleanses the scalp and removes excess oil and buildup.

30. Castor Oil and Oatmeal Facial Scrub

Ingredients:

2 tablespoons of castor oil.

2 tablespoons of finely milled oats.

1 tablespoon honey.

Preparation:

In a dish, blend the castor oil, ground oats, and honey until thoroughly incorporated.

Gently massage the scrub into moist skin in circular strokes for 1-2 minutes.

Allow the ingredients to enter the skin by leaving the scrub on for an extra 5 minutes. Rinse with lukewarm water, then pat dry.

Benefits:

Castor oil thoroughly hydrates and nourishes the skin, making it supple and moisturized.

Oatmeal gently exfoliates dead skin cells, resulting in a smoother, brighter complexion.

Honey contains antimicrobial qualities that assist to combat acne and inflammation.

31. Castor Oil and Papaya Hair Mask

Ingredients:

1/2 ripe papaya.

2 tablespoons of castor oil.

1 tablespoon of coconut oil.

Preparation:

Mash the ripe papaya in a dish until smooth. Mix in the castor and coconut oils with the crushed papaya.

Apply the mixture to moist hair, concentrating on the scalp and strands.

After 30-45 minutes of using the mask, properly rinse with shampoo and water.

Benefits:

Castor oil stimulates hair growth and strengthens follicles.

Papaya includes enzymes that assist to eliminate buildup from the scalp and unclog hair follicles.

Coconut oil hydrates and nourishes hair, making it smooth and lustrous.

32. Castor Oil and Matcha Green Tea Face Mask

Ingredients:

1 tablespoon of castor oil.

1 tablespoon matcha green tea powder.

1 spoonful of plain yogurt.

Preparation:

In a dish, blend the castor oil, matcha green tea powder, and yogurt until thoroughly incorporated.

Use the mixture on clean, dry skin, avoiding the eyes.

For the next 15 to 20 minutes, Leave the mask onRinse with lukewarm water, then pat dry.

Benefits:

Castor oil intensively hydrates and nourishes the skin, resulting in a healthy complexion.

Matcha green tea contains antioxidants, which help protect the skin from environmental harm and prevent inflammation.

Yogurt contains lactic acid, which gently exfoliates the skin and brightens and evens out its tone.

33. *Castor Oil and Cinnamon Lip Plumper*

Ingredients:

1 tablespoon of castor oil.

1/2 a teaspoon of crushed cinnamon

1/2 teaspoon of coconut oil.

Preparation:

In a small mixing bowl, blend the castor oil, ground cinnamon, and coconut oil well.

Apply a thin coating of the mixture to your lips, concentrating on the lip line and any areas you wish to plump.

Leave it on for 5-10 minutes, then rinse with lukewarm water.

Apply a hydrating lip balm next.

Benefits:

Castor oil gently hydrates and nourishes the lips, leaving them smooth and moisturized.

Cinnamon stimulates blood flow to the lips, making them momentarily expand and seem larger.

Coconut oil increases hydration and helps to lock in moisture, avoiding dryness.

34. Castor Oil and Seaweed Body Wrap

Ingredients:

2 tablespoons of castor oil.

1/4 cup powdered seaweed.

1/4 cup warm water.

Preparation:

In a dish, combine the castor oil, powdered seaweed, and warm water to produce a thick paste.

Apply the mixture to your body, concentrating on areas with cellulite or dry skin.

Wrap your body with plastic wrap or a towel and leave for 30-60 minutes.

Rinse in the shower with warm water.

Benefits:

Castor oil penetrates deeply into the skin, hydrating and nourishing it from the inside.

Seaweed is high in vitamins, minerals, and antioxidants, which help cleanse and enhance skin look.

The body wrap firms and tones the skin, decreasing the appearance of cellulite and improving general skin health.

35. *Castor Oil and Rose Water Facial Toner.*

Ingredients:

2 tablespoons of castor oil.

1/4 cup rose water.

1 tablespoon of witch hazel.

Preparation:

In a clean container, add castor oil, rose water, and witch hazel.

Close the bottle and shake vigorously to combine all of the contents properly.

After cleaning your face, apply the toner with a cotton pad and gently brush it over your skin.

Let it dry before adding moisturizer.

Benefits:

Castor oil hydrates and nourishes the skin, making it smooth and moisturized.

Rose water has anti-inflammatory qualities that assist in soothing inflamed skin and minimize redness.

Witch hazel serves as an astringent, constricting pores and regulating oil production.

36. Castor Oil and Lemon Foot Scrub

Ingredients:

2 tablespoons of castor oil.

1/4 cup granulated sugar.

Zest from 1 lemon

1 tablespoon of lemon juice.

Preparation:

In a bowl, blend the castor oil, granulated sugar, lemon zest, and lemon juice until thoroughly incorporated.

Wet your feet and apply the scrub, concentrating on tough regions such as heels and soles.

Massage in gentle circular strokes for a few minutes.

Rinse with warm water, then pat dry.

Benefits:

Castor oil hydrates and softens dry, cracked heels, resulting in smooth, healthy feet.

Sugar exfoliates dead skin cells, resulting in softer, brighter skin.

Citric acid in lemon juice can help exfoliate dead skin cells and brighten dark spots.

37. Castor Oil and Shea Butter Body Butter

Ingredients:

2 tablespoons of castor oil.

2 tablespoons of shea butter.

1 tablespoon cocoa butter.

1 tablespoon of coconut oil.

5 drops of vanilla extract (optional).

Preparation:

In a double boiler, combine the shea butter, cocoa butter, and coconut oil over low heat.

Once melted, remove from heat and allow it to cool slightly.

Mix in the castor oil and vanilla extract (if using).

Transfer the mixture to a clean container and let it harden.

Benefits:

Castor oil significantly hydrates the skin, making it smooth and moisturized.

Shea and cocoa butter are high in vitamins and antioxidants, which nourish and moisturize the skin.

Coconut oil adds hydration and helps to retain moisture, leaving the skin soft and smooth.

38. Castor Oil and Rosemary Hair Rinse

Ingredients:

2 tablespoons of castor oil.

1/4 cup dried rosemary leaves.

2 glasses of water.

Preparation:

Heat the water in a small saucepan until it boils.

Add the dried rosemary leaves to the boiling water and allow it to simmer for 10-15 minutes.

Strain the rosemary-infused water into a basin and allow it to cool somewhat.

Stir in the castor oil until well blended.

Apply the combination as a last rinse after washing and conditioning your hair.

Benefits:

Castor oil benefits the scalp and encourages healthy hair development.

Rosemary improves blood circulation in the scalp, which promotes hair development and prevents hair loss.

The hair rinse improves shine and suppleness while relaxing the scalp and decreasing dandruff.

39. Castor Oil and Honey Hair Mask

Ingredients:

2 tablespoons of castor oil.

1 tablespoon of raw honey.

1 egg yolk.

Preparation:

In a dish, blend the castor oil, raw honey, and egg yolk until thoroughly incorporated.

Apply the mixture to damp hair, beginning at the roots and progressing to the ends.

Cover your hair with a shower cap and let the mask sit for 30-60 minutes.

Rinse thoroughly with lukewarm water and apply shampoo as normal.

Benefits:

Castor oil benefits the scalp and encourages healthy hair development.

Honey hydrates and softens the hair, making it easier to handle and less likely to break.

Egg yolk includes protein and vitamins that help to build and brighten your hair.

35.   *Castor Oil and Rose Water Facial Toner*

Ingredients:

2 tablespoons of castor oil.

1/4 cup rose water.

1 tablespoon of witch hazel.

Preparation:

In a clean container, add castor oil, rose water, and witch hazel.

Close the bottle and shake vigorously to combine all of the contents properly.

After cleaning your face, apply the toner with a cotton pad and gently brush it over your skin.

Let it dry before adding moisturizer.

Benefits:

Castor oil hydrates and nourishes the skin, making it smooth and moisturized.

Rose water has anti-inflammatory qualities that assist in soothing inflamed skin and minimize redness.

Witch hazel serves as an astringent, constricting pores and regulating oil production.

36. Castor Oil and Lemon Foot Scrub

Ingredients:

2 tablespoons of castor oil.

1/4 cup granulated sugar.

Zest from 1 lemon

1 tablespoon of lemon juice.

Preparation:

In a bowl, blend the castor oil, granulated sugar, lemon zest, and lemon juice until thoroughly incorporated.

Wet your feet and apply the scrub, concentrating on tough regions such as heels and soles.

For a few minutes, and in circular strokes Massage gentle

Rinse with warm water, then pat dry.

Benefits:

Castor oil hydrates and softens dry, cracked heels, resulting in smooth, healthy feet.

Sugar exfoliates dead skin cells, resulting in softer, brighter skin.

Citric acid in lemon juice can help exfoliate dead skin cells and brighten dark spots.

37. Castor Oil and Shea Butter Body Butter

Ingredients:

2 tablespoons of castor oil.

2 tablespoons of shea butter.

1 tablespoon cocoa butter.

1 tablespoon of coconut oil.

5 drops of vanilla extract (optional).

Preparation:

In a double boiler, combine the shea butter, cocoa butter, and coconut oil over low heat.

Once melted, remove it from the heat and allow it to cool slightly.

Mix in the castor oil and vanilla extract (if using).

Transfer the mixture to a clean container and let it harden.

Benefits:

Castor oil significantly hydrates the skin, making it smooth and moisturized.

Shea and cocoa butter are high in vitamins and antioxidants, which nourish and moisturize the skin.

Coconut oil adds hydration and helps to retain moisture, leaving the skin soft and smooth.

38. Castor Oil and Rosemary Hair Rinse

Ingredients:

2 tablespoons of castor oil.

1/4 cup dried rosemary leaves.

2 glasses of water.

Preparation:

Until the water in a saucepan boils continue heating up

Add the dried rosemary leaves to the boiling water and allow it to simmer for 10-15 minutes.

Strain the rosemary-infused water into a basin and allow it to cool somewhat.

Stir in the castor oil until well blended.

Apply the combination as a last rinse after washing and conditioning your hair.

Benefits:

Castor oil benefits the scalp and encourages healthy hair development.

Rosemary improves blood circulation in the scalp, which promotes hair development and prevents hair loss.

The hair rinse improves shine and suppleness while relaxing the scalp and decreasing dandruff.

39. Castor Oil and Honey Hair Mask

Ingredients:

2 tablespoons of castor oil.

1 tablespoon of raw honey.

1 egg yolk.

Preparation:

In a dish, blend the castor oil, raw honey, and egg yolk until thoroughly incorporated.

Apply the mixture to damp hair, beginning at the roots and progressing to the ends.

For the next 30-60 minutes, let the mask sit, and also Cover your hair with a shower cap

Rinse thoroughly with lukewarm water and apply shampoo as normal.

Benefits:

Castor oil benefits the scalp and encourages healthy hair development.

Honey hydrates and softens the hair, making it easier to handle and less likely to break.

Egg yolk includes protein and vitamins that help to build and brighten your hair.

40. Castor Oil and Turmeric Face Mask

Ingredients:

1 tablespoon of castor oil.

1 teaspoon of turmeric powder.

1 spoonful of yogurt

Preparation:

In a small bowl, combine the castor oil, turmeric powder, and yogurt until smooth.

Use the mixture on clean, dry skin, avoiding the eyes.

For the next 15 to 20 minutes, Leave the mask on

Rinse with lukewarm water, then pat dry.

Benefits:

Castor oil intensely hydrates and nourishes the skin, making it smooth and supple.

Turmeric contains anti-inflammatory and antioxidant qualities that assist in lightening skin and minimizing acne.

Lactic acid in yogurt gently exfoliates the skin and helps to erase dark patches and discoloration.

41. Castor Oil and Aloe Vera Hair Conditioner.

Ingredients:

2 tablespoons of castor oil.

2 teaspoons of aloe vera gel.

1 tablespoon of coconut oil.

Preparation:

In a dish, blend the castor oil, aloe vera gel, and coconut oil until well-mixed.

Apply the mixture to moist hair, concentrating on the ends.

After 20-30 minutes, rinse completely with water.

Benefits:

Castor oil benefits the scalp and encourages hair development.

Aloe vera includes enzymes that heal dead skin cells on the scalp and serve as a natural conditioner for hair.

Coconut oil enters the hair shaft to moisturize and prevent damage.

42. Castor Oil and Bentonite Clay Face Mask

Ingredients:

1 tablespoon of castor oil.

1 spoonful of bentonite clay.

1 tablespoon of apple cider vinegar.

Preparation:

In a mixing bowl, combine the castor oil, bentonite clay, and apple cider vinegar until smooth.

Use the mixture on clean, dry skin, avoiding the eyes.

For the next 10-15 minutes and until it begins to dry Leave the mask on

Rinse with lukewarm water, then pat dry.

Benefits:

Castor oil hydrates and nourishes the skin, which reduces dryness and flakiness.

Bentonite clay absorbs excess oil and pollutants from the skin, therefore detoxifying and clarifying pores.

Apple cider vinegar regulates the skin's pH and reduces irritation and redness.

43.Castor Oil and Coffee Scrub

Ingredients:

2 tablespoons of castor oil.

2 tablespoons of finely ground coffee.

1 tablespoon of brown sugar.

1 tablespoon of coconut oil.

Preparation:

In a bowl, blend the castor oil, finely powdered coffee, brown sugar, and coconut oil until thoroughly incorporated.

Wet your skin and massage the scrub in circular strokes, concentrating on cellulite or dry regions.

Massage for a few minutes and then rinse with warm water.

Pat dry and apply moisturizer.

Benefits:

Castor oil significantly hydrates the skin, making it smooth and moisturized.

Coffee grinds exfoliate dead skin cells, resulting in smoother, firmer skin.

Brown sugar helps exfoliation, while coconut oil delivers moisture and nutrition.

44. Castor Oil and Tea Tree Oil Acne Treatment Serum

Ingredients:

2 tablespoons of castor oil.

5-6 drops of Tea Tree essential oil

1 tablespoon of jojoba oil.

Preparation:

In a tiny dropper bottle, mix the castor oil, tea tree essential oil, and jojoba oil.

Close the bottle and shake vigorously to combine the ingredients.

After cleaning your face, dab a few drops of the serum over the afflicted areas.

Gently massage in circular strokes until completely absorbed.

Benefits:

Castor oil regulates oil production and reduces the irritation linked with acne.

Tea tree essential oil contains antibacterial qualities that help eliminate acne-causing germs and prevent outbreaks.

Jojoba oil hydrates the skin without blocking pores, keeping it balanced and moisturized.

45. *Castor Oil and Yogurt Hair Mask*

Ingredients:

2 tablespoons of castor oil.

1/2 cup of plain yogurt.

1 tablespoon honey.

Preparation:

In a dish, stir the castor oil, yogurt, and honey until completely incorporated.

Apply the mixture to damp hair, beginning at the roots and progressing to the ends.

For the next 30-60 minutes, let the mask sit, and also Cover your hair with a shower cap

Rinse thoroughly with lukewarm water and apply shampoo as normal.

Benefits:

Castor oil benefits the scalp and encourages healthy hair development.

Yogurt contains lactic acid, which cleanses the scalp and removes dead skin cells.

Honey moisturizes the hair, making it softer and more manageable.

46. Castor Oil and Orange Peel Body Scrub

Ingredients:

2 tablespoons of castor oil.

1/4 cup of dried orange peel powder.

1/4 cup granulated sugar.

1 tablespoon of coconut oil.

Preparation:

In a bowl, blend the castor oil, orange peel powder, granulated sugar, and coconut oil until thoroughly mixed.

Wet your skin and massage the scrub in circular strokes, concentrating on rough regions such as elbows and knees.

Massage for a few minutes and then rinse with warm water.

Pat dry and apply moisturizer.

Benefits:

Castor oil intensely hydrates the skin, making it smooth and supple.

Orange peel powder removes dead skin cells, revealing smoother, brighter skin.

Coconut oil promotes moisture and nutrition, while sugar gently exfoliates.

47. *Castor Oil and Avocado Hair Serum*

Ingredients:

2 tablespoons of castor oil.

1/2 ripe avocado.

1 tablespoon of argan oil.

Preparation:

In a mixing basin, mash the ripe avocado until completely smooth.

Mix in the castor and argan oils with the mashed avocado.

Apply serum to damp hair, concentrating on the mid-lengths and ends.

Leave it on for 30-60 minutes, then thoroughly rinse with water.

Benefits:

Castor oil benefits the scalp and encourages hair development.

Avocado is high in vitamins and fatty acids, which nourish and strengthen the hair.

Argan oil enhances gloss and repairs damaged hair, making it silky and manageable.

48: Castor Oil and Green Tea Eye Serum

Ingredients:

1 tablespoon of castor oil.

1 tablespoon brewed green tea, chilled.

1 teaspoon of vitamin E oil.

Preparation:

In a small dish, blend the castor oil, brewed green tea, and vitamin E oil until thoroughly mixed.

Transfer the mixture to a clean dropper bottle for convenient administration.

Apply a tiny quantity of serum to the under-eye region with your fingertips.

Pat gently until completely absorbed.

Benefits:

Castor oil nourishes and hydrates the sensitive skin beneath the eyes, minimizing the appearance of fine lines and wrinkles.

Green tea contains antioxidants, which assist to reduce puffiness and brighten the under-eye region.

Vitamin E oil nourishes and protects the skin, resulting in a young and vibrant appearance.

49. Castor Oil and Lemon Hair Rinse

Ingredients:

Ingredients: 2 tablespoons castor oil, 1 lemon juice.

2 glasses of water.

Preparation:

in a bowl the lemon juice and Castor oil Should be combined

Dilute the mixture with two glasses of water.

After washing and conditioning, apply the diluted mixture to your hair as a final rinse.

Massage it gently into your scalp and hair, then rinse well with lukewarm water.

Benefits:

Castor oil benefits the scalp and encourages healthy hair development.

Lemon juice removes excess oil and buildup from the scalp, leaving the hair feeling clean and fresh.

Lemon juice's acidic characteristics also assist in sealing the hair cuticles, leaving it smoother and shinier.

50. Castor Oil and Mint Foot Cream

Ingredients:

2 tablespoons of castor oil.

1/4 cup Shea butter

1 tablespoon of coconut oil.

5 drops peppermint essential oil.

Preparation:

In a double boiler, combine the shea butter and coconut oil over low heat.

Allow it to cool slightly after removing it from the heat source once it has melted

Mix in the castor oil and peppermint essential oil.

Transfer the mixture to a clean container and let it harden.

Benefits:

Castor oil profoundly hydrates and nourishes dry, cracked heels, resulting in softer, smoother feet.

Shea butter and coconut oil give substantial hydration, replenishing moisture to dry, rough skin.

Peppermint essential oil provides a cooling action that relieves sore feet while leaving a delightful smell.

51. Castor Oil and Banana Hair Smoothie

Ingredients:

One ripe banana.

2 tablespoons of castor oil.

1/4 cup coconut milk.

1 tablespoon honey.

Preparation:

In a blender, mix the ripe banana, castor oil, coconut milk, and honey.

Blend until smooth and creamy.

Apply the mixture to damp hair, beginning at the roots and progressing to the tips.

Place a shower cap over your hair and leave it on for 30-60 minutes.

Rinse thoroughly with lukewarm water and apply shampoo as normal.

Benefits:

Castor oil benefits the scalp and encourages healthy hair development.

Bananas are high in potassium, vitamins, and natural oils, which help smooth and condition hair.

Coconut milk and honey provide hydration and luster to the hair, making it velvety smooth, and manageable.

52. Castor Oil and Lavender Bath Bombs

Ingredients:

1 cup baking soda.

1/2 cup citric acid.

1/2 cup cornstarch.

2 tablespoons of castor oil.

10-15 drops of lavender essential oil.

Dried lavender blossoms (optional).

Witch hazel (in a spray bottle)

Preparation:

Combine the baking soda,cornstarch and baking soda In a large bowl

In a separate small basin, mix the castor oil and lavender essential oil.

Slowly pour the oil mixture into the dry ingredients, stirring constantly.

If desired, add dried lavender flowers and thoroughly combine.

Spray the mixture with witch hazel, a little at a time, until it holds together when pressed.

Pack the mixture into bath bomb molds and allow to dry overnight.

Carefully take the bath bombs from the molds and keep them in an airtight container.

Benefits:

Castor oil hydrates and nourishes the skin, making it smooth and moisturized.

Lavender essential oil offers relaxing effects that help relax the body and mind, resulting in a good night's sleep.

These bath bombs create a luxury spa-like experience, leaving your skin feeling pampered and invigorated.

53. Castor and Rosemary Scalp Massage Oil.

Ingredients:

2 tablespoons of castor oil.

1 tablespoon of olive oil.

5 drops of rosemary essential oil.

Preparation:

In a small dish, combine castor oil, olive oil, and rosemary essential oil.

Place the bowl in hot water or microwave for a few seconds to warm up the mixture.

Section your hair and apply the oil mixture straight to the scalp.

Massage the scalp in circular strokes for 5-10 minutes to improve circulation.

Leave the oil on for at least 30 minutes, or overnight for further conditioning.

Shampoo and condition your hair as normal.

Benefits:

Castor oil nourishes the scalp and stimulates hair growth by increasing blood circulation.

Olive oil moisturizes the scalp and softens the hair, which reduces dryness and flakiness.

Rosemary essential oil stimulates hair follicles, which promotes new growth and prevents hair loss.

54. *Castor and Chamomile Face Cleansing Oil.*

Ingredients:

2 tablespoons of castor oil.

2 teaspoons of grapeseed oil.

3 drops of chamomile essential oil

Preparation:

In a tiny container, mix the castor oil, grapeseed oil, and chamomile essential oil.

Close the bottle and shake vigorously to combine the ingredients.

Apply a tiny quantity of cleaning oil to your face and gently massage it into the skin.

Soak a washcloth in warm water and put it over your face for a few seconds.

Use the washcloth to gently remove oil and pollutants from your skin.

If desired, use a light cleaner afterward.

Benefits:

Castor oil thoroughly cleanses the skin by dissolving debris, makeup, and excess oil without removing natural moisture.

Grapeseed oil is lightweight and non-comedogenic, thus it is excellent for all skin types. It aids in balancing oil production and preventing breakouts.

Chamomile essential oil contains anti-inflammatory and relaxing characteristics that help to relieve irritated skin and decrease redness.

55. Castor Oil and Coconut Milk Hair Mask

Ingredients:

2 tablespoons of castor oil.

1/4 cup coconut milk.

1 tablespoon honey.

1 teaspoon of vanilla essence.

Preparation:

In a mixing bowl, blend the castor oil, coconut milk, honey, and vanilla extract until well incorporated.

Apply the mixture to moist hair, concentrating on the roots and tips.

For the next 30-60 minutes, let the mask sit, and also Cover your hair with a shower cap

Rinse thoroughly with lukewarm water and apply shampoo as normal.

Benefits:

Castor oil benefits the scalp and encourages healthy hair development.

Coconut milk contains vitamins and minerals that nourish and strengthen the hair.

Honey gives hydration and gloss to the hair, while vanilla extract imparts a delicious fragrance.

56. Castor Oil and Cucumber Eye Gel

Ingredients:

1 tablespoon of castor oil.

1/4 cucumber, peeled and chopped.

1 tablespoon of aloe vera gel.

Preparation:

Blend the chopped cucumbers until smooth.

Pour the cucumber juice through a fine mesh strainer to remove the liquid.

In a small dish, blend the castor oil, cucumber juice, and aloe vera gel until well-mixed.

Place the mixture in a clean container for storage.

Benefits:

Castor oil hydrates and nourishes the sensitive skin around the eyes, minimizing the appearance of fine lines and wrinkles.

Cucumber juice has a cooling effect, which helps to minimize puffiness and dark circles under the eyes.

Aloe vera gel soothes and moisturizes the skin, giving it a fresh and renewed appearance.

57. *Castor Oil and Grapefruit Lip Scrub*

Ingredients:

1 tablespoon of castor oil.

1 tablespoon of granulated sugar.

1 teaspoon of grapefruit zest.

1 teaspoon honey.

Preparation:

In a small bowl, blend the castor oil, granulated sugar, grapefruit zest, and honey until thoroughly incorporated.

Gently scrape the mixture onto your lips in circular movements for 1-2 minutes.

Rinse with warm water, then pat dry.

use lip balm,To keep your lips moisturized

Benefits:

Castor oil profoundly hydrates and nourishes the lips, making them soft and smooth.

Granulated sugar exfoliates dead skin cells, resulting in softer, plumper lips.

Grapefruit zest contains vitamin C, which brightens and rejuvenates the lips, while honey provides moisture.

58. *Castor Oil and Clay Scalp Detox Mask*

Ingredients:

2 tablespoons of castor oil.

1 spoonful of bentonite clay.

1 tablespoon of apple cider vinegar.

1 tablespoon of water.

Preparation:

In a mixing dish, combine the castor oil, bentonite clay, apple cider vinegar, and water until smooth.

Apply the mixture to your scalp, then separate your hair as required.

For the next 15 to 20 minutes, the mask Should be left on

Rinse thoroughly with lukewarm water and apply shampoo as normal.

Benefits:

Castor oil nourishes the scalp and stimulates hair growth while also removing impurities and buildup.

Bentonite clay detoxifies the scalp by removing impurities and excess oil, leaving it clean and revitalized.

Apple cider vinegar balances the scalp's pH levels and regulates oil production, creating a healthy scalp environment.

59. *Castor Oil and Almond Oil Hair Serum*

Ingredients:

2 tablespoons of castor oil.

1 tablespoon of almond oil.

5 drops of rosemary essential oil.

Preparation:

In a small bowl, mix the castor oil, almond oil, and rosemary essential oil.

Mix thoroughly until all of the ingredients are equally combined.

Transfer the mixture to a clean dropper bottle for convenient administration.

Apply a few drops of serum to your scalp and gently massage it.

Let it sit overnight or for at least 30 minutes before shampooing.

Benefits:

Castor oil promotes hair development and provides the scalp with important nutrients.

Almond oil is high in vitamin E, which stimulates hair follicles and encourages healthy hair development.

Rosemary essential oil increases blood circulation to the scalp, which promotes hair development and prevents hair loss.

CONCLUSION

Castor oil is a versatile component that provides several advantages for supporting healthy living, with a special emphasis on smoothing skin and improving the look of lashes and eyebrows.

When used topically, castor oil profoundly moisturizes the skin, keeping it smooth and supple and preventing the production of fine lines and wrinkles. Its hydrating characteristics make it great for treating under-eye bags and puffiness while also regenerating the fragile skin in this area.

Adding castor oil to lashes and brows with a clean mascara wand helps stimulate hair follicles, resulting in stronger, healthier growth over time. Its mild yet powerful cleaning characteristics make it an ideal choice for removing makeup, leaving the skin clean and invigorated without eliminating its natural oils.

By including castor oil into your daily skincare regimen, you may get smoother skin, thicker lashes, and more defined brows, which will improve your overall look and promote a healthier lifestyle.

THANK YOU PAGE

Thank you for selecting this book. Your support is really appreciated. Similarly, I am grateful for the purchase of this book.

Your input is valuable; please share your ideas in a review. It serves as a reference for future improvements. Enjoy reading and utilizing it!